Natural Strategies for Varicose Veins Management

César González Andrade

Natural Strategies for Varicose Veins Management

Supplements, Nutrients and Alternative Therapies for the Prevention and Treatment of Varicose Veins and Venous Ulcers

César González Andrade

At the time of publication of this book, the articles that were referenced are available for free under the Creative Commons (CC BY) license. This license allows others to distribute, remix, adapt, and develop the content of the articles, including for commercial purposes, if they are given credit for the original creation. Neither the authors nor the editors participated in the creation of this book, but their results served for the research of the topics discussed here. In the bibliography you can find the accreditation of their articles.

Warning

Health sciences, like nutrition, are constantly changing fields, therefore, the information contained here may vary. This book is for informational purposes and the information presented should not be considered as a substitute for a medical prescription, diagnosis, or treatment. The author cannot be held liable for any damage caused by omitting this warning. It is always recommended to consult a doctor or nutritionist.

Index

Introduction

Varicose veins and chronic venous insufficiency are conditions that affect millions of people worldwide, causing not only pain and discomfort, but also cosmetic problems that can affect quality of life. For those who suffer from these conditions, the search for effective and natural solutions can be a path full of frustrations and disappointments. This book is presented as a comprehensive and accessible guide for those looking to address varicose veins from a holistic perspective, combining nutrition, supplementation, and alternative therapies.

In "Natural Strategies for the Management of Varicose Veins," we explore a variety of essential nutrients, supplements, and herbal treatments that have been shown to be effective in the management and prevention of varicose veins and venous ulcers. Each chapter of this book is carefully designed to provide information based on scientific research, clinical experiences, and traditional practices that have stood the test of time.

From Omega-3s and their role in venous health, to the power of Centella Asiatica and Ginkgo Biloba, we will discover together how these nutrients and medicinal plants can become indispensable allies in your fight against varicose veins. We will also address the impact of physical activity, the importance of body weight balance, and specific strategies to improve venous health in the work environment.

This book not only focuses on the physical aspect of venous disease, but also recognizes the importance of a comprehensive approach that includes the mind and spirit. Practices such as yoga and meditation are presented as complementary tools for stress management and improved circulation, demonstrating that total well-being is possible through a multifaceted approach.

As you delve into these pages, you will find not only valuable information, but also hope and motivation. This book is written for you, who are looking for a natural and effective solution to your venous problems. Whether you are a patient, a healthcare professional, or just someone interested in improving your well-being, "Natural Strategies for Managing Varicose Veins" will provide you with the tools and knowledge needed to take control of your vein health in an informed and initiative-taking way.

Let me accompany you on this journey to a life with less pain, more vitality, and optimal venous health. I am convinced that, with the right information and strategies, you can achieve a better quality of life and say goodbye to varicose veins finally. Let us start this path to full and natural venous health together!

Omega-3s and their Role in the Management of Varicose Veins

Have you ever wondered how something as small as an oil capsule can influence problems as complex as varicose veins? In this chapter, we will explore the role that long-chain omega-3 fatty acids (LCn3) play in cardiovascular health and, more specifically, in varicose veins, those visible, dilated veins that can appear primarily in the legs.

Omega-3 fatty acids are known for their ability to improve cardiovascular health, but did you know that they could also have a role in managing varicose veins?

Omega-3s play a crucial role in modulating blood lipid levels. They can help lower serum triglycerides and slightly increase HDL (the "good" cholesterol). These changes in lipid profiles are beneficial for maintaining a healthy cardiovascular system and, in the context of varicose veins, could help prevent complications associated with poor circulation.

One of the lesser-known, but equally important, benefits of Omega-3s is their ability to function as anti-inflammatories. This is especially relevant if you suffer from ulcers associated with varicose veins. Recent studies have shown that Omega-3 supplementation resulted in significant reductions in the length, width, and depth of ulcers. In addition, these fatty acids improved insulin sensitivity and reduced levels of C-reactive protein (CRP), an inflammatory marker. The typical dosage for these benefits is 1000 mg twice daily.

For groups with specific needs, such as people who are pregnant or breastfeeding, or those taking blood-thinning medications, medical supervision is crucial before starting Omega-3 supplementation due to the risk of drug interactions and side effects such as bleeding complications.

Instead of focusing only on supplements, I encourage you to consider including foods naturally rich in Omega-3 in your diet. Fatty fish such as salmon, mackerel, and sardines, as well as nuts and seeds, are not only excellent sources of Omega-3s, but they also offer a wide range of other essential nutrients that supplements cannot provide. These whole foods help support a balanced diet and healthy lifestyle, crucial for managing varicose veins.

Practical Tips for Omega-3 Ingestion

1. Diversify Your Sources: Incorporate a variety of Omega-3 sources into your diet, including fatty fish such as salmon and sardines, as well as chia seeds and walnuts.

2. Healthy Cooking: Prepare your fish baked or grilled instead of fried to preserve essential fatty acids and avoid unhealthy fats.

3. Quality Supplements: If you opt for Omega-3 supplements, look for those certified for their purity and free of contaminants such as mercury.

How much Omega-3 do I need daily?

 The recommended dosage may vary, but between 250 mg and 1000 mg of EPA and DHA combined daily is suggested for healthy adults.

Can Omega-3 supplements interact with other medications?

Yes, especially with blood thinners. Omega-3s can increase the risk of bleeding, so it is crucial to consult with a doctor before starting supplementation if you are taking medications like Warfarin.

Can vegetarians get enough Omega-3s?

Vegetarians can opt for plant sources such as flax seeds, chia seeds, and walnuts, or supplements derived from algae.

Tips for Medical Supervision

If you decide to take Omega-3 supplements, it is advisable to have regular checkups to monitor your overall cardiovascular health and adjust doses if necessary.

Report any adverse effects, such as fish-tasting burps, upset stomach, or allergic reactions, to your doctor.

Make sure your doctor evaluates your entire diet and lifestyle to properly adjust any Omega-3 supplements in the context of your overall health.

Conclusion

Although long-chain omega-3s do not directly fix varicose veins, their impact on overall health and microcirculation can be a vital component in your management strategy. Are you ready to make a slight change to your diet that could have a significant impact on your quality of life?

Evaluation of Zinc Sulfate in the Treatment of Venous Ulcers

Have you ever felt that frustration when following a treatment that does not offer the expected results? In this chapter, we will delve into the evaluation of zinc sulfate, a proposed treatment for venous ulcers, taking a close look at its effectiveness and relevance for people like you who are dealing with varicose vein complications.

Zinc plays a critical role in numerous biological processes, including collagen synthesis and immune function, both of which are essential in the wound healing process. However, when it comes to venous ulcers, the story is more complex than it might seem at first glance.

Through studies that have varied in methodology, from doses of 440 to 660 mg per day and treatment durations of four weeks to one year, attempts have been made to determine the efficacy of zinc sulfate in the healing of venous ulcers. Interestingly, the results have shown no statistically significant differences between zinc sulfate treatment and control groups, whether placebo or no treatment.

Based on the available evidence, it is recommended to consider zinc sulfate alone as an adjunctive treatment, after evaluating other methods that are more effective and better supported by scientific research. It is crucial to understand that although zinc is vital for numerous biological processes, its supplementation has not been shown to be a definitive solution for venous ulcers.

Measurement of serum zinc levels has been part of the evaluation in several studies, revealing the importance of monitoring these levels to properly adjust dosage and avoid misinterpretations that could affect the effectiveness of treatment.

Although essential for collagen synthesis and immune function, zinc supplementation has not shown a clear advantage in the healing rate of venous ulcers, suggesting that adequate levels of zinc are necessary, but not sufficient on their own to ensure healing.

Safety Considerations in the Use of Zinc Sulfate

Studies have reported that the side effects of zinc sulfate are mild, including symptoms such as constipation, nausea, and rashes. However, it is critical to be vigilant for these effects, especially in patients who may be taking high doses or who have pre-existing conditions that are likely to worsen.

Practical Tips for Using Zinc Sulfate

1. opt for high-quality zinc sulfate supplements, which are certified for their purity to ensure effectiveness and minimize risks of contaminants.

2. Consider creams or gels containing zinc sulfate to apply directly to venous ulcers, following the manufacturer's instructions to avoid irritation or adverse reactions.

How much zinc sulfate can I take daily for varicose veins?

The dosage may vary, but it is recommended not to exceed 440 mg to 660 mg per day. It is essential to follow your doctor's recommendations to adjust the dosage to your specific needs.

Can zinc sulfate interact with other medications?

Yes, zinc sulfate can interact with certain antibiotics and rheumatoid arthritis medications, reducing their absorption. Always consult with your doctor before combining treatments.

What foods are rich in zinc?

Oysters, red meat, poultry, beans, and nuts are excellent sources of zinc. Integrating these foods into your diet can help maintain optimal levels without the need for excessive supplementation.

It is important to perform blood tests periodically to monitor zinc levels in your body, adjusting supplementation as needed to avoid toxicity or deficiency.

Report any new or worsening symptoms, such as nausea or rashes, to your doctor immediately to assess the need to adjust your treatment.

If you are considering increasing your zinc intake through diet, a consultation with a nutritionist can provide a balanced eating plan that meets your nutritional needs without exceeding safe zinc limits.

Conclusion: Thinking About the Future

While zinc sulfate has been explored as a treatment option, evidence for its effectiveness is limited and should be carefully evaluated compared to other, more established treatment options. In the next chapter we will learn about a benefit of Zinc.

With these recommendations, we hope you feel more prepared to discuss with your doctor the treatment options that are best suited for you. Are you ready to make informed decisions that optimize your varicose vein well-being and management?

Nutritional and Dermatological Strategies for the Comprehensive Management of Varicose Veins with Zinc

Imagine feeling a constant itch in your legs, a symptom that not only makes you uncomfortable, but also keeps you awake at night. Now imagine discovering that this discomfort may be related not only to visible varicose veins but also to your skin's hydration status and zinc levels in your body. This chapter is dedicated to exploring this connection and offering practical recommendations based on recent findings.

Varicose veins not only affect the circulation and aesthetics of your legs, but they can also significantly impact the health of your skin. Aspects such as stratum corneum hydration and trans epidermal water loss (TEWL) are critical to maintaining the integrity of the skin barrier, and these factors may be compromised in people with varicose veins.

The data reveals that people with varicose veins and itching tend to have noticeably lower levels of hydration in the stratum corneum, which can exacerbate itching and discomfort. This deterioration in the skin barrier is a critical factor that we need to address. It is crucial to monitor skin hydration in patients with varicose veins. Regular use of moisturizers can improve hydration and offer significant relief.

An elevated TEWL is indicative of a compromised skin barrier, which can increase dryness and itching. It is advised to periodically evaluate TEWL for any deterioration in skin barrier integrity and take corrective action.

Importance of Zinc in Skin Function

Not only is zinc crucial for skin integrity and immune function, but zinc levels have also been found to be significantly lower in people with varicose veins and itching. Consider zinc supplementation under medical supervision, especially if blood tests show deficiencies. This can improve not only skin hydration but also reduce TEWL.

Practical Application for Daily Improvement

Use of Moisturizers: Regular application of moisturizers is essential to keep the skin hydrated and strengthen the skin barrier.

Zinc Supplementation: Be sure to check zinc levels and adjust supplementation as needed to optimize skin health benefits.

Medical care for patients with varicose veins should integrate dermatologic evaluations along with vascular treatment. This multidisciplinary collaboration between dermatologists, angiologists, and nutritionists is vital to address all aspects of varicose veins holistically.

Practical Tips for Varicose Veins Management and Skin Health

1. Choosing and Applying Moisturizers

opt for creams that contain components such as hyaluronic acid and ceramides that help retain moisture in the skin.

Apply moisturizer after showering when skin is still slightly damp to maximize absorption.

How much zinc should I take to improve skin health?

The recommended amount of zinc varies, but a range of 11-22 mg daily is suggested for adults, depending on individual needs and medical supervision.

What other nutrients are important for skin health in people with varicose veins?

In addition to zinc, vitamins such as C and E are crucial for their antioxidant properties that protect the skin and improve its elasticity.

Regular Consultations

Schedule regular visits with your doctor to monitor zinc levels
and adjust dosing as needed. This is especially important if
you are using zinc supplements.

Integrated Dermatological Evaluations

Consider regular evaluations with a dermatologist to compre-
hensively address the skin aspects of varicose veins and adjust
treatment accordingly.

This comprehensive approach not only addresses the skin
symptoms associated with varicose veins, but also aims to improve the patient's overall quality of life by managing often-
overlooked complications. Are you ready to adopt these practices into your daily routine and observe improvements not
only in your varicose veins but also in the overall health of
your skin?

By understanding and applying these recommendations, you
can take an active role in managing your varicose veins, significantly improving both your physical well-being and your per-
sonal satisfaction with the treatment.

Magnesium Key Nutrient for Ulcer Healing in Varicose Veins Patients

Have you ever felt that, despite your efforts, managing varicose veins seems like a never-ending road? Not only do varicose veins affect the aesthetics of your legs, but they can also be complicated by venous ulcers, a challenge that requires not only medical treatment but also nutritional support. In this chapter, we will explore how vitamin E and magnesium can play a crucial role in your recovery.

When we talk about varicose veins and especially venous leg ulcers (VLU), nutrition can have a direct and significant impact on the speed and effectiveness of healing. Recent research has highlighted the role of certain nutrients, such as vitamin E and magnesium, which are essential not only for maintaining good health but also for facilitating specific processes that can speed up recovery from varicose vein-associated ulcers.

Vitamin E and Magnesium: Allies in Healing

Vitamin E, known for its antioxidant properties, along with magnesium, which regulates inflammatory processes, have

shown promising results in supplementation for the treatment
of venous ulcers.

The combination of 250 mg of magnesium oxide and 400 IU
of vitamin E taken daily has been shown to significantly reduce ulcer size, improve glycosylated hemoglobin (HbA1c)
levels, and optimize lipid profiles. These nutrients work by improving endothelial function and reducing oxidative stress,
which in turn facilitates ulcer healing.

Clinical Supervision:

Given the potential of these nutrients to exceed the tolerable
upper intake limit (TUIL) for magnesium, medical supervision
is essential. Supplementation should be supervised by professionals to monitor for any adverse effects and adjust doses as
needed. This tracking ensures that the benefits of supplementation are maximized without compromising your safety.

Are you using all available resources to manage your varicose
veins and associated complications? Incorporating these nutrients into your daily regimen under medical supervision could
be a transformative step toward better health and quality of
life.

Practical Application: Beyond Theory

Supplement Use: Consider talking to your doctor about including vitamin E and magnesium supplements in your diet. This is not only a preventative measure, but also an accelerator in the healing of venous ulcers.

Regular Monitoring: Make sure your progress with these supplements is monitored regularly to adjust dosage and address any concerns that may arise.

Comprehensive Approach: Nutrition and Medical Treatment

Integrating nutritional management with established medical treatment offers a holistic strategy that addresses not only varicose veins and their symptoms but also underlying conditions such as venous ulcers. This collaboration between nutritionists and doctors is essential to ensure effective and safe treatment.

1. Safety and Dosage of Supplements:

Vitamin E: The mentioned dose of 400 IU daily is within safe limits for most adults. However, it is essential to consider that high doses of vitamin E can interact with certain medications and increase the risk of bleeding, especially in people taking blood thinners.

Magnesium: The 250 mg dose of magnesium oxide is typically safe, but it is important to monitor the effects, as high doses can cause problems such as diarrhea or electrolyte imbalances.

Medical supervision is crucial to adjust the dosage and prevent complications.

2. Effectiveness and Mechanisms of Action:

Vitamin E and magnesium have well-documented roles in reducing oxidative stress and improving endothelial function. However, direct evidence for its efficacy in venous ulcer healing is limited and mixed. The combination of both for this specific purpose is not widely studied, so although promising, it should be considered experimental.

3. Evidence-Based Recommendations:

Given the potential for benefits and risks, it is prudent for vitamin E and magnesium supplementation to be done under medical supervision. This is especially important for people with pre-existing conditions or who are taking other medications.

4. Integration into the Treatment Strategy:

Integrating these supplements into the treatment plan may offer additional benefits in terms of cardiovascular health and ulcer healing. However, it should be part of a broader approach that includes other medical treatments and lifestyle changes.

This analysis confirms that the inclusion of vitamin E and magnesium in the management of venous ulcers should be done carefully, evaluating each case individually. Medical supervision is essential to ensure that supplementation is safe and effective, adjusting to the specific needs of the patient and their clinical context.

Practical Tips for Vitamin E and Magnesium Supplementation

1. Initiation of Supplementation

Before starting any supplement regimen, especially vitamin E and magnesium, consult with your doctor to make sure it is right for your specific needs, especially if you are taking other medications.

What foods are rich in vitamin E and magnesium?

Vitamin E is found in foods such as almonds, spinach, and vegetable oils. Magnesium is present in nuts, seeds, legumes, and whole grains.

How do I know if I need more vitamin E or magnesium in my diet?

Symptoms such as muscle cramps, irritability, and wound healing difficulties may indicate a deficiency. However, it is essential to perform blood tests to determine your exact levels.

Tips for Medical Supervision

Regular Consultations

 Schedule regular blood tests to monitor your vitamin E and magnesium levels. Adjust your supplementation based on these results and your doctor's recommendations.

Drug Interaction Management

 Vitamin E may interact with blood thinners and other medications. Discuss these potential interactions with your doctor to avoid complications.

This comprehensive approach not only improves treatment outcomes, but also empowers the patient to take an active role in their health. With the right knowledge and the right support, the road to recovery can be more efficient and less painful. Are you ready to take the next step in your care and recovery?

Horse Chestnut Extract: A Natural Ally in the Treatment of Varicose Veins

Have you ever felt that your legs not only look affected by varicose veins, but also experience pain, swelling and an annoying itching sensation? If so, this chapter will offer you a refreshing perspective on how horse chestnut seed extract (HSEC) can be a vital ally in your fight against these symptoms.

Horse chestnut extract is not just a folk remedy; is a scientifically supported treatment for chronic venous insufficiency (CVI). Controlled research has shown its ability to relieve symptoms such as leg pain, edema, and pruritus, transforming not only the appearance of the legs, but also significantly improving the quality of life of those affected.

Clinical Evidence of HCSE Benefit

1. Leg Pain Relief:

EHSC has shown a significant reduction in pain in several studies. For example, an average reduction of 42.40 mm in the visual analog scale indicates a marked improvement in leg pain.

2. Reduction of Edema:

Studies reveal that HCSE is effective in reducing edema, with an improvement measured in a 40.10 mm reduction in the edema scale, compared to placebo.

3. Treatment of CVI-Associated Pruritus:

In addition to reducing edema and pain, HCSE has also been shown to be effective against pruritus, significantly improving this irritating symptom.

4. Leg Circumference Management:

Treatment with HCSE has managed to reduce the circumference of the leg, facilitating both aesthetic and functional improvement in patients.

Biological Mechanisms Behind EHSC

Venous Strengthening: HCSE contains aescin, a component that strengthens vein walls, improves venous tone, and reduces capillary permeability.

Reduced Inflammation: In addition, it is suggested that HCSE moderates local inflammation, which helps relieve itching and other inflammatory symptoms.

Practical Application: How to Use the EHS

Recommended Dose: The effective dosage of HCSE is 100-150 mg daily, standardized to escin. It is vital to begin any supplementation under medical supervision to adjust the dosage according to your response and needs.

Monitoring Side Effects: Although well tolerated, it is crucial to be on the lookout for potential side effects, especially gastrointestinal ones.

Integrating EHSC with other treatment modalities such as compression stockings and lifestyle changes can offer you a holistic and effective approach to managing chronic venous insufficiency. This natural treatment not only relieves physical symptoms, but also improves your overall well-being, allowing you to resume daily activities with less discomfort and more confidence.

Monitoring and Security Considerations:

Although EHCH is well tolerated, it is important to monitor patients for any side effects, especially those related to the gastrointestinal system. The most common side effects include gastrointestinal discomfort, but they are usually mild.

It is recommended to integrate the HCSE into a larger treatment plan that may include compression stockings and lifestyle adjustments. Medical supervision is crucial to tailor dosage and treatment to each patient's individual needs, thus ensuring maximum effectiveness and safety.

Practical Tips for Using the EHSC

1. Start of Supplementation:

Check with your doctor before starting HCSE, especially if you are taking other medications that may interact.

Can I use HCSE while I am taking blood-thinning medications?

You should consult with your doctor before using HCSE if you are on blood thinning treatment, because of the potential for increased risk of bleeding.

What should I do if I experience side effects with HCSE?

If you experience side effects such as gastrointestinal discomfort, it is important to let your doctor know to adjust your dosage or review other treatment options.

Tips for Medical Supervision

Regular Evaluation:

It is crucial to get regular checkups to assess how HCSE affects your body, especially if you have pre-existing conditions that could be affected by its use.

Dose Adjustment:

Based on your response to treatment and lab test results, your doctor can adjust the dose to maximize efficacy and minimize risks.

Optimizing the Management of Chronic Venous Insufficiency with Centella Asiatica

In the constant search for effective solutions for the complications of chronic venous insufficiency (CVI) and venous microangiopathy, nature offers a powerful ally: the total triterpene fraction of Centella asiatica (TTFCA). This chapter is dedicated to exploring how this plant, used for centuries in traditional medicine, is now emerging as a promising treatment according to recent scientific evidence.

Discovering Centella Asiatica

Imagine walking down a quiet path, encountering a plant that is not only capable of beautifying the landscape, but also possesses the power to relieve some of the most persistent and painful discomforts of varicose veins. Centella asiatica, known for its healing properties, has been extensively studied in clinical settings to validate its benefits in the treatment of CVI.

Proven Efficacy in CVI Symptoms

1. General Symptom Improvement:

Rigorous studies have shown that TTFCA significantly improves CVI symptoms, such as edema, leg pain, and pruritus.

Effective doses: TTFCA dosage has ranged from 30 mg twice daily to 120 mg daily, depending on the severity of symptoms, with treatments lasting between 28 and 60 days.

2. Impact on Microcirculation and Leg Volume:

TTFCA has shown remarkable improvements in leg volume and ankle and calf circumference, contributing to an effective reduction in edema.

It also improves microcirculatory parameters, including transcutaneous partial pressure of oxygen and carbon dioxide (tcPO2, tcPCO2), and venous response (VAR).

Safety and Tolerability

Although the adverse effects associated with TTFCA are mild, such as stomach pain and nausea, their incidence is low, reinforcing the safety profile of this treatment.

Biological Mechanisms of Action

Strengthening the Capillary Barrier: TTFCA reduces capillary permeability by strengthening the venous walls, which decreases leakage and edema formation.

Improved Microcirculation: It acts directly on improving venous flow, thus facilitating venous return, and reducing blood stagnation in the lower extremities.

Practical Application and Comprehensive Management

Adjusted Administration: It is recommended to initiate treatment with dosing based on symptom severity and adjust based on individual patient response.

The total triterpene fraction of Centella asiatica (TTFCA) has been extensively investigated for its effect on improving the symptoms of chronic venous insufficiency (CVI), showing promising results in various investigations. TTFCA has been shown to significantly improve common symptoms of CVI such as edema, leg pain, and pruritus. These improvements have been observed with doses ranging from 30 mg twice daily to 120 mg daily, applied for periods ranging from 28 to 60 days.

As for the safety and tolerability of TTFCA, studies have indicated that side effects are mild and may include gastrointestinal symptoms such as stomach pain and nausea, although these are rare. This favorable safety profile makes TTFCA an option to consider in the management of CVI.

It is important that any TTFCA supplementation be supervised by a healthcare professional to customize the dose to individual needs and responses, and to ensure proper integration with other forms of CVI management, such as compression therapy and other dermo protective treatments. This ensures a comprehensive approach that maximizes therapeutic benefits while minimizing the risk of adverse effects.

Before you start taking TTFCA, check with a healthcare professional to make sure it is right for you, especially if you are taking other medications.

How long should I take TTFCA to see improvements in CVI symptoms?

Studies suggest taking TTFCA for a period of 28 to 60 days to see significant improvements in CVI symptoms, but the duration can vary depending on individual response.

Are there any side effects to taking TTFCA?

Side effects are mild and include gastrointestinal symptoms such as stomach pain and nausea. If you experience adverse effects, it is important to consult a doctor.

Monitoring Effects and Dose Adjustments:

It is vital that TTFCA dosing is personalized and monitored by a physician, especially at the start of treatment, to adjust doses based on patient needs and responses.

Comprehensive Evaluation:

Consider regular leg circumference and skin quality assessments to monitor the effectiveness of TTFCA in managing CVI and adjust treatment as needed.

Conclusion

The total triterpene fraction of Centella asiatica is presented as a valuable therapeutic option to improve symptoms and quality of life in patients with CVI. With documented benefits and a favorable safety profile, this natural treatment deserves to be seriously considered in chronic venous insufficiency management protocols, always under the supervision of health professionals and tailored to the patient's individual needs.

The Importance of Vitamin D in the Healing of Varicose Vein-Associated Ulcers

Have you ever wondered why some wounds heal more slowly than others, especially when it comes to leg ulcers associated with varicose veins? Through this chapter, we will explore how an essential nutrient, vitamin D, plays a crucial role in healing these ulcers, giving you a new perspective and tools to better manage your health.

The Vital Role of Vitamin D in Your Body

Vitamin D, known as the "sunshine vitamin," is not only critical for keeping your bones strong, but it also has a significant impact on other areas of your health, including immune system function and inflammatory processes. This essential nutrient helps regulate your body's response to infection and inflammation, two critical factors in ulcer healing.

How Vitamin D Supports Ulcer Healing

1. Improved Immune Function:

Vitamin D is vital for the proper functioning of your immune system. It helps activate your body's defenses that fight infection, which is essential for effective ulcer healing.

2. Modulation of Inflammation:

In addition, this vitamin plays a role in modulating the inflammatory response. By controlling inflammation, vitamin D can reduce tissue damage in the ulcer area, thus facilitating healing.

Recommended Dosage and Observed Benefits

Effective Dosage:The recommended dosage for seeing improvements in ulcer healing is 4,000 IU of vitamin D weekly. This amount has been shown to be effective in significantly improving healing.

Impact on biochemical parameters: Not only are improvements observed in ulcer healing, but also in important biochemical parameters such as HbA1c (an indicator of blood glucose control) and lipid profile, which includes cholesterol and triglycerides, thus improving cardiovascular health.

Correlation Between Vitamin D Levels and Ulcer Healing

A positive correlation has been found between adequate vitamin D levels and improved ulcer healing. This means that maintaining optimal vitamin D levels is not only beneficial for your bone and immune health, but also essential for recovering more quickly from venous ulcers.

Practical Tips for Vitamin D Ingestion

1. Absorption Optimization:

Take vitamin D with a meal that contains fat. Vitamin D is fat-soluble, so its absorption is improved when ingested with foods rich in healthy fat, such as avocado, nuts, seeds, or olive oil.

2. Diversification of Sources:

Do not rely solely on supplements; try to get vitamin D from natural sources as well. Salmon, tuna, herring, and eggs are excellent sources, as are fortified products such as some types of milk and cereals.

3. Regularity and Measurement:

Take vitamin D supplements regularly as recommended by your doctor and consider regular blood tests to monitor your vitamin D levels, adjusting the dosage if necessary.

1. How much vitamin D should I take daily if I have varicose veins?

The dosage may vary depending on individual needs and health status. For ulcer healing, up to 4,000 IU has been used weekly, but it is vital to consult a doctor for a personalized dose.

2. Can I get enough vitamin D from the sun alone?

Sun exposure can help produce vitamin D, but the amount varies depending on geographic location, season, and skin type. In many cases, especially in less sunny climates, it is necessary to supplement with diet or supplements.

3. What do I do if I experience side effects with vitamin D supplements?

If you experience side effects such as stomach pain, fatigue, or symptoms of excess calcium (confusion, increased thirst), see your doctor immediately.

Tips for Medical Supervision

1. Initial Consultation and Regular Evaluations:

Before starting any supplement, especially if you have pre-existing conditions, it is crucial to get a medical evaluation. Regular follow-ups will help adjust the dose and avoid interactions with other medications.

2. Interaction Monitoring:

Tell your doctor about all medications and supplements you are taking to avoid interactions, especially if you are using medications that affect blood clotting or the metabolism of other nutrients.

3. Education on Signs of Toxicity:

Although rare, vitamin D toxicity can occur, especially with high doses. It is important to be informed about signs of toxicity, such as nausea, vomiting, weakness, and kidney problems, and to know when to seek medical help.

Conclusion

Integrating a nutritional approach, especially increasing vitamin D intake, could be a valuable strategy in your treatment plan for varicose veins and their complications. Discuss with your doctor the possibility of measuring your vitamin D levels and consider supplementation if necessary to optimize your healing process and improve your quality of life.

This chapter has equipped you with key insights into how a simple adjustment to your vitamin regimen could translate into significant improvements in your skin's health and faster ulcer healing. I invite you to take active steps toward more effective recovery and improved well-being. Are you ready to make that change?

Vitamin C in the Management of Varicose Veins: Beyond Cardiovascular Prevention

Imagine a clear, sunny day, perfect for a walk in the park, but you stop, worried about the pain and swelling in your legs due to varicose veins. Could a simple change in your diet or daily vitamin C supplementation be the key to improving your quality of life? In this chapter, we will explore how vitamin C, beyond its known benefits, can be an ally in the management of varicose veins.

Vitamin C is recognized for its powerful antioxidant effect and its role in cardiovascular health. However, recent studies have shown that although vitamin C does not directly reduce the risk of cardiovascular diseases such as heart attacks or strokes, no significant negative effects of its supplementation have been found on overall vascular health. This could be relevant for you if you have varicose veins, as maintaining good cardiovascular health is essential in their management.

Biological Mechanisms of Vitamin C in Vascular Health

1. Vitamin C protects your body's cells from damage caused by free radicals through its antioxidant function. This process is crucial for maintaining the integrity of your blood vessel walls, which is especially relevant for people with varicose veins.

2. Although it does not directly reduce major cardiovascular disease events, vitamin C improves the microvascular environment. This is important for managing symptoms associated with varicose veins, such as inflammation and pain, through its influence on local blood circulation and the reduction of oxidative stress.

Role in Collagen Synthesis:

Vitamin C is essential for the synthesis of collagen, the protein responsible for the strength and elasticity of the skin and blood vessels. This is especially relevant in the context of ulcers that can develop in people with advanced varicose veins.

In studies, vitamin C levels have been observed to be significantly lower in patients with diabetic ulcers, suggesting a potential role in its prevention and management.

Practice

In the absence of firm evidence to support exclusive vitamin C supplementation to prevent cardiovascular events, it is advisable to obtain this vitamin through a diet rich in fruits and vegetables, such as citrus fruits, strawberries, kiwi, peppers, and broccoli.

If you decide to supplement, it is essential to do so under the supervision of a health professional. This is crucial, especially if you have pre-existing cardiovascular or circulatory health conditions.

This chapter invites you to consider vitamin C not just as a supplement, but as part of a healthy lifestyle that could significantly improve your management of varicose veins and their associated complications.

Practical Tips for Vitamin C Supplementation

1. Increase your intake of foods rich in vitamin C such as citrus fruits, strawberries, kiwi, peppers, and broccoli. Including these foods in your daily diet can improve the quality of your skin and strengthen your blood vessels.
2. Consider supplementation only under the guidance of a healthcare professional, especially if you have pre-existing conditions or are taking other medications.

Can vitamin C directly improve varicose veins?

Vitamin C does not directly treat varicose veins, but it improves vascular health and blood vessel integrity through its antioxidant effects, which can help manage symptoms associated with varicose veins.

How much vitamin C is safe to consume daily?

The recommended amount of vitamin C for adults varies, but 65 to 90 mg daily is sufficient. It is important not to exceed 2,000 mg daily to avoid side effects.

Regular Consultations:

Schedule regular checkups with your doctor to monitor the effectiveness of vitamin C supplementation and adjust the dosage if necessary.

Drug Interaction Evaluation:

Discuss with your doctor all medications you are taking to ensure there are no adverse interactions with vitamin C supplementation.

The Balance of Body Weight and Varicose Veins: A Crucial Balance

As a nutritionist dedicated to the study and application of holistic wellness strategies, I have repeatedly observed how weight management directly influences the treatment and symptoms of varicose veins. In this chapter, I invite you to explore not only the scientific connections between being overweight and varicose veins but also how practical adjustments in your daily life can significantly improve your venous health.

Think of the veins in your legs as roads that, under extra pressure, become prone to obstruction and damage. Overweight and obesity, which affect 64% of certain populations, put considerable pressure on these "highways", intensifying varicose vein symptoms and increasing the risk of serious complications such as venous ulcers. But how exactly does this happen?

Excess weight not only physically burdens the veins, but also causes metabolic and inflammatory changes. For example, obesity increases intra-abdominal pressure, which hinders venous return, which is essential for healthy blood flow. In addition, excess adipose tissue secretes substances that promote a chronic inflammatory state, further complicating the health of your veins.

48

Innovations in the Treatment of Varicose Veins for Different Body Mass Indexes

Thermal Endo venous Therapy (ETA), a modern and effective technique, has proven to be particularly effective, closing almost 100% of the treated trunk veins, regardless of whether the patient has a high or normal BMI. Despite its high efficacy, post-treatment follow-up reveals that complications, although rare, tend to be more frequent in people with a higher BMI, highlighting the need for careful monitoring and personalized adjustments in the management of anticoagulation and pain after the procedure.

Practical Strategies for a Healthy Weight

Reducing and maintaining a healthy weight not only improves your venous profile, but also boosts the effectiveness of treatments such as ETA. The combination of a balanced, nutrient-dense, low-processed diet, along with a regular exercise regimen that supports circulation, can transform your varicose vein management. Consulting a nutritionist can provide you with a personalized plan that fits your specific needs and goals.

Reflect on how each daily choice affects your vascular health. Are you ready to take proactive steps to relieve your symptoms and improve your quality of life? Implementing these recommendations will not only benefit you in the short term but will also help you avoid future complications associated with varicose veins.

Practical Tips

Incorporation of Moderate Physical Activity:

Integrate daily walks of at least 30 minutes to improve circulation and relieve pressure in the veins of the legs. Gradually increase the duration and intensity according to your ability.

Leg Raise Exercises:

Perform leg raise exercises twice a day to facilitate venous return. These may include lying down and lifting your legs against a wall for 5 to 10 minutes.

Maintaining Proper Hydration:

Drink between 1.5 and 2 liters of water a day to help maintain good circulation and reduce bloating.

How does being overweight affect varicose veins?

Being overweight increases pressure in the veins in your legs, which can weaken your venous valves and exacerbate varicose veins.

What type of exercise is recommended for someone with varicose veins?

Prefer low-impact exercises such as swimming, walking, or biking, and avoid activities that require jumping or running on hard surfaces.

Tips for Medical Supervision

Initial Consultation with a Health Care Professional: Before modifying your diet or starting a new exercise regimen, consult with a doctor to ensure that the activities selected are safe for you.

Regular Progress Monitoring: Schedule regular follow-up visits to assess progress and make necessary adjustments to your varicose vein management plan.

Nutritional Evaluation by a Specialist: Consider consulting a dietitian to develop a meal plan that supports vascular health, tailored to your specific nutritional needs.

This chapter has been an invitation to look beyond conventional varicose vein treatment, delving into how a comprehensive approach, including weight management, can significantly improve your treatment outcomes and overall well-being. Your journey to recovering from and maintaining varicose veins is deeply tied to your lifestyle, and every step you take toward a healthy weight is a step toward healthier veins.

Physical Activity and Nutrition for the Management of Varicose Veins

In our journey to a healthier life, especially for those facing challenges like varicose veins, the balance between proper physical activity and optimal nutrition is critical. This chapter focuses on how physical activity, combined with compression therapy, plays a crucial role in the treatment and prevention of varicose veins and their complications, such as venous ulcers.

Imagine your veins as rivers that need a constant flow to stay clean and functional. When we lead a sedentary lifestyle, it is as if those rivers stagnate, which can aggravate conditions like varicose veins. This is where physical activity comes into play. Performing low-impact exercises such as walking or swimming can significantly improve blood circulation, crucial for preventing blood stagnation in the veins. But how exactly does it work?

Physical activity stimulates circulation in the lower extremities, improving oxygenation and nutrient transport to the affected areas, which accelerates the healing of ulcers.

Regular exercise can moderate the systemic inflammatory response associated with varicose veins and venous ulcers.

Nitric Oxide (NO) Metabolism Enhancement: Exercise increases the production of NO, essential for vasodilation and vascular health.

Recommendations Based on the Review of Physical Activity Effectiveness

Through a rigorous analysis of studies, I have identified that physical activity, especially when combined with compression therapy, can markedly improve the healing of venous ulcers, and prevent their recurrence. The exercises should be low-cost, easy to implement and adapted to the ability of everyone.

Practical Implementation of Physical Activity

1. Multicomponent Exercise Programs:

Combine resistance training with foot and ankle mobility exercises. These interventions should be monitored to ensure proper execution and improve clinical outcomes.

2. Supervision and Support:

Implement remote monitoring or virtual training, particularly useful in situations such as the COVID-19 pandemic, to maintain adherence to exercise programs.

3. Continuous Evaluation:

To monitor the effects of physical activity on ulcer healing and to assess quality of life, pain levels and associated economic costs.

Practical Tips

Establish a Regular Exercise Routine:

Start with low-impact activities such as walking or swimming, and gradually increase the duration and frequency of exercises. Consider including cycles of foot and ankle exercises to improve venous return.

Integrate Stretching Sessions:

Include stretching routines in your exercise program. This can help improve flexibility and circulation, reducing pressure in the veins.

Wearing Compression Stockings During Exercise:

Wear compression stockings during and after exercise to improve venous support and reduce the risk of swelling.

What type of exercises are most effective for varicose veins?

Low-impact exercises such as walking, swimming, and cycling are the most recommended to improve circulation without putting too much pressure on the veins.

How does compression therapy combine with exercise help?

Compression therapy helps improve blood flow and reduces swelling, while exercise promotes healthy blood circulation and can prevent the progression of varicose veins.

Regular Consultation with Professionals:

Schedule regular visits with your doctor to monitor the progression of varicose veins and adjust treatment as needed. This is crucial especially after starting a new exercise regimen.

Evaluation of the Adequacy of Compression Stockings:

Make sure that the compression stockings are the right size and compression. A specialist can help you select the most suitable type for your condition.

Monitoring Exercise Response:

Observe how your body reacts to exercise and report any new symptoms or increased symptoms to your doctor.

Conclusion: A Step Forward in the Treatment of Varicose Veins

Although the specifics of optimal physical activity are yet to be determined, incorporating moderate exercise as an adjunct to compression therapy may offer additional benefits in the management of varicose veins and venous ulcers. This chapter not only underlines the importance of a comprehensive strategy that combines both treatments, but also encourages the personalization and adaptation of these recommendations to the individual needs of each patient, thus guaranteeing maximum efficacy and safety in their application.

As you consider this information, reflect on how you can integrate these tips into your daily life. What steps can you take today to activate your circulation and strengthen your veins? This holistic approach not only improves your venous condition, but also elevates your overall well-being, allowing you to enjoy a more active and healthy life.

Yoga and its Impact on Varicose Veins Management

Have you ever stopped to consider that an ancient practice like yoga could be effective not only for your overall mental and physical well-being, but also for combating varicose veins? This chapter breaks down the findings of a groundbreaking study on the effects of yoga on varicose veins, explaining how it could be integrated into your daily routine to significantly improve your vascular health.

The study in question took a comprehensive look at the effects of yoga on people with varicose veins, focusing on several key aspects:

1. Reduced Inflammatory Markers: Participants who practiced yoga showed a significant decrease in levels of high-sensitivity C-reactive protein (hs-CRP) and homocysteine (HCy), crucial indicators of inflammation in the body.

2. Improvement in Physical and Cardiovascular Parameters: Notably, the yoga group experienced reductions in body weight, body mass index (BMI), blood pressure, and heart rate, suggesting a positive cardiovascular impact of this practice.

3. Influence on Microcirculation: The intervention with yoga improved the function of the calf muscle and venous return, vital elements to combat venous stasis that frequently accompanies varicose veins.

Study-Based Recommendations

Adopting Yoga Regimens: Incorporating yoga into the treatment of varicose veins can markedly improve circulation and reduce markers of inflammation. Regular sessions, tailored to everyone, can make a significant difference in vascular health.

Continuous Monitoring of Cardiovascular Parameters: It is recommended to closely monitor blood pressure and heart rate to assess response to treatment and adjust yoga practice as needed.

Regular Assessment of Endothelial Function: Regular testing for inflammatory markers is crucial, which can provide insights into the evolution and management of varicose veins.

Biological Mechanisms Underlying the Benefits of Yoga

Calf Muscle Function and Venous Return: Yoga strengthens calf muscle function, facilitating venous return and reducing the likelihood of varicose veins forming.

Reduced Systemic Inflammation: Relaxation techniques and yoga poses help mitigate stress and inflammation, positively affecting veins and overall vascular health.

Improved Microcirculation: Yoga practices encourage better blood circulation, crucial for managing varicose veins and reducing symptoms such as pain and swelling.

Practical Application and Specific Context

Personalization of Treatment: It is essential to adapt yoga sessions to the abilities and limitations of each person, ensuring that everyone can participate safely and effectively.

Ongoing Education and Support: Providing ongoing information and support to patients is key to overcoming physical and psychological barriers, such as fear of pain or concern for safety.

Conclusion: Yoga, a Valuable Complement to the Treatment of Varicose Veins

Including yoga as part of an integrated approach to varicose vein management is not only beneficial for physical health, but also improves quality of life by reducing pain and inflammation. This chapter has walked you through yoga's potential to transform your varicose vein management, underscoring the importance of a personalized, well-supervised approach.

Are you ready to take the next step and explore how yoga can help you live better with varicose veins? Consider this practice not just exercise, but an essential part of your journey to optimal vascular health.

Practical Tips

1. Yoga Poses Beneficial for Varicose Veins:

Integrate poses such as "leg against the wall" (Viparita Karani) and "bridge pose" (Setu Bandhasana) into your daily practice.

These poses help improve blood circulation in the legs, relieving venous pressure and reducing swelling.

2. Frequency and Duration:

Practice yoga at least three times a week for 30 to 45 minutes per session.

Regular practice improves flexibility, strengthens the calf muscles, and promotes efficient venous return.

3. Combine Yoga with Self-Care Measures:

Wear compression stockings during the day and perform gentle stretches every few hours.

This helps maintain good circulation and prevent the formation of new varicose veins.

Can yoga really help improve varicose veins?

Yes, yoga can be beneficial for people with varicose veins. Yoga poses and breathing techniques improve blood circulation, reduce inflammation, and strengthen the calf muscles, which facilitates venous return and decreases the symptoms of varicose veins.

What is the best yoga poses for varicose veins?

Some of the most effective poses include "leg against the wall" (Viparita Karani), "bridge pose" (Setu Bandhasana), and "downward facing dog pose" (Adho Mukha Svanasana). These poses help improve circulation and reduce pressure in the veins in your legs.

Is it safe to practice yoga if I already have advanced varicose veins?

Yes, but it is important to do so under the supervision of a qualified yoga instructor and preferably with the consent of your doctor. Adapting postures and avoiding those that put too much pressure on the veins is crucial to avoid complications.

Tips for Medical Supervision

1. Initial Consultation:

Before starting any yoga program, consult with your doctor to evaluate your venous condition and receive specific recommendations.

This ensures that the chosen yoga poses are safe and suitable for your situation.

2. Regular Monitoring:

Schedule regular checkups with your doctor to monitor your progress and adjust your yoga plan as needed.

Continuous monitoring helps identify improvements and adjust the intensity or frequency of the practice to maximize benefits without risk.

3. Collaboration with Yoga Instructors:

Let your yoga instructor know about your varicose vein condition so they can adapt poses and offer safe modifications.

A knowledgeable instructor can provide you with a personalized practice that respects your limitations and promotes your well-being.

Conclusion

Yoga is not only a beneficial practice for the mind and body, but it can also be a powerful tool in managing varicose veins. Integrating yoga into your daily routine, under proper supervision, can significantly improve your vascular health, reduce inflammation, and relieve symptoms associated with varicose veins. Are you ready to explore how yoga can transform your varicose vein management and improve your quality of life?

Strategies to Improve Venous Health in the Workplace

Imagine a typical day at your workplace, how many hours do you spend sitting or standing in a fixed position? Did you know that this simple routine can significantly influence the health of your veins? In this chapter, we will explore how slight changes in your work habits can have a profound impact on the prevention and management of varicose veins, a condition that affects millions of people each year.

Recent studies have shown that the prevalence of venous ulcers in advanced stages is higher in individuals who remain standing for more than four hours at a time. This data is crucial because it highlights how the work routine can contribute to the development of serious venous problems.

When we remain in a static position, whether standing or sitting, the blood circulation in our legs is negatively affected. This occurs because prolonged inactivity prevents the action of the 'muscle pump' in our calves, which is essential for pushing blood back to the heart. Without this pumping action, blood can pool in the veins, increasing venous pressure and, over time, contributing to the development of varicose veins.

Practical Adaptations in the Work Environment

1. Alternating between standing and sitting:

Introduce regular intervals where you switch between sitting and standing. If your job involves a long time in one position, take short breaks to walk or do light stretching.

Not only does this habit reduce the pressure in the veins in your legs, but it also promotes better blood circulation.

2. Redesign of the work environment:

  Strategy: Adjust workspaces to facilitate mobility. For example, setting up areas for employees to perform simple stretches or walk for a few minutes.

These modifications can make a significant difference in the venous health of everyone in the work environment.

Clinical Evaluation and Referral to Specialists

If symptoms of chronic venous insufficiency are detected, prompt evaluation by a specialist is essential. Diagnostic tests can range from non-invasive methods, such as Doppler ultrasound, to more complex techniques. However, for the comfort and safety of patients, non-invasive testing is preferred.

Prevention and Ongoing Care

In sectors where standing days are the norm, such as in commerce and health, implementing preventive measures is essential. This may include:

Wearing compression stockings: They help improve circulation and prevent blood pooling in the veins.

Low-impact activities: Walking programs or light exercise during breaks can be significantly beneficial.

Practical Tips

Adopt an Ergonomic Workstation: Make sure your workspace allows you to alternate between sitting and standing. Consider investing in adjustable desks that facilitate this alternation.

Set Reminders to Move: Use alarms or apps that remind you to take regular breaks to stretch or walk, which can help improve circulation and reduce venous pressure.

Customize Your Stretching Routine: Include specific exercises you can do at work to improve circulation, such as rotating your ankles, flexing your calf muscles, and stretching your legs.

How long should I stand to avoid varicose vein problems if my work is mostly sedentary?

Ideally, try to get up at least 5 minutes every hour to reduce the risk of varicose veins and other circulatory problems.

What kind of compression stockings are recommended for someone who is on their feet all day?

Look for well-fitting graduated compression stockings that have the level of compression recommended by your doctor, usually between 20 and 30 mmHg for work situations.

Tips for Medical Supervision

Regular Consultation with a Specialist: If you are at risk of developing varicose veins or already have them, it is important to have regular checkups with a vascular specialist who can monitor your progress and adjust your treatment plan as needed.

Professional Compression Stocking Evaluation: Make sure a healthcare professional helps you choose and adjust your compression stockings to ensure they are providing proper support without compromising circulation.

Symptom Monitoring: Report any new symptoms or increased symptoms to your doctor, such as increased swelling, changes in skin color, or leg pain.

Conclusion: Acting in Our Hands

Every step you take, every change you make to your work routine not only improves your venous health, but also enhances your overall quality of life. Are you ready to transform your work environment and take care of your veins with the same dedication with which you take care of your work?

This chapter has provided you with practical tools and essential knowledge so that you can make informed decisions about how to best manage varicose veins in the work context. Remember, every little action counts on your path to optimal venous health.

The Power of Ruscus Aculeatus in the Treatment of Varicose Veins

In a world where nature offers remedies for all our ailments, a little-known but powerful plant stands out for its ability to relieve the symptoms of varicose veins: Ruscus aculeatus, commonly known as "butcher's broom." Throughout this chapter, we will explore how this plant can transform your approach to managing varicose veins, relying on a solid scientific basis to ensure effectiveness and safety.

Imagine a small perennial shrub, hardy and full of secrets. Native to Europe, Ruscus aculeatus is more than just a plant: it is an arsenal of bioactive components including saponins such as ruscogenin and neoruscogenin, flavonoids, sterols, and triterpenes. These compounds are not just complicated names; They are the keys to revitalizing tired and overloaded veins.

Benefits of Microcirculation

1. Venotonic Activity:

What does this mean? Ruscus aculeatus improves venous tone. It works by stimulating the release of norepinephrine, a neurotransmitter that activates adrenergic receptors in the walls of the veins, causing them to tighten and shrink in diameter, which helps propel blood to the heart.

Practical Benefit: By improving venous tone, the feeling of heaviness in the legs is reduced and the progression of varicose veins is prevented.

2. Endothelial Protection:

How does it work? The plant exhibits powerful antioxidant and anti-inflammatory effects, protecting the cells that line the inside of the veins. This is crucial for preventing vascular damage and maintaining healthy blood circulation.

Clinical Use and Safety

Proven Effectiveness: Ruscus aculeatus has been shown to be effective in the treatment of peripheral venous disease (PVD) and hemorrhoids. Studies show a significant reduction in the diameter of the affected veins, which relieves symptoms and improves the quality of life of patients.

Adverse Effects: Although well tolerated, it is crucial to be aware of possible adverse effects. One case reported diabetic ketoacidosis, underscoring the need for medical supervision when including this supplement in your regimen.

Adverse Effects and Safety:

The side effects mentioned are mild, such as constipation or nausea. However, the isolated case of reported diabetic ketoacidosis requires caution and medical supervision, especially in patients with risk factors or pre-existing conditions. This underscores the importance of medical supervision when considering supplementation with Ruscus aculeatus.

Recommendations for Safe and Effective Use

Dosage and Administration: The typically recommended dosage varies, but studies suggest that doses of 100-150 mg daily are effective. It is crucial to follow dosage instructions and consult a healthcare professional before starting any new supplementation, especially to adjust the dosage based on individual response and prevent interactions or side effects.

Medical Monitoring and Supervision: Given the potential for side effects and interaction with other medical conditions, monitoring by a healthcare professional is essential. This ensures that the treatment is not only effective but also safe for the patient.

Practical Tips

Regular Use of Extracts: Consider incorporating Ruscus aculeatus supplements into your daily routine. The recommended dose is usually 100-150 mg daily, depending on the concentration of the extracts and the medical recommendation.

Topical Applications: Explore topical products containing Ruscus aculeatus, such as gels or creams, which can be applied directly to affected areas to relieve symptoms such as heaviness and edema.

Combination with Other Treatments: Use Ruscus aculeatus in combination with other treatments such as compression stockings and dietary adjustments to maximize the benefits in managing varicose veins.

Is Ruscus aculeatus suitable for all patients with varicose veins?

Although beneficial for many, its use should be evaluated individually, especially in people with pre-existing health conditions. Always consult a professional before starting any new supplement.

How long should it take for Ruscus aculeatus to see improvements?

The benefits can typically be seen after a few weeks of continuous use. However, results may vary depending on the individual and the severity of symptoms.

Tips for Medical Supervision

Initial Evaluation and Follow-up: Before starting treatment with Ruscus aculeatus, it is important to perform a medical evaluation to determine the suitability of this supplement for your specific case. Regular follow-up will help adjust the dose and monitor the efficacy and safety of the treatment.

Monitoring Interactions and Side Effects: Since Ruscus aculeatus can interact with other medications and supplements, medical supervision is crucial to prevent adverse interactions and recognize any side effects early.

Conclusion: A Green Ally for Your Veins

Ruscus aculeatus is not just a supplement; It is nature's promise for better vein health. By integrating this plant into your varicose vein management strategy, accompanied by regular exercise and a balanced diet, you can achieve significant control over your symptoms and improve your quality of life. This chapter has broken down not only how the plant works for your benefit, but also how you can implement it safely and effectively.

Hawthorn (Crataegus spp.) and its Role in Varicose Vein Management

Imagine a plant that not only beautifies the landscape with its delicate flowers and red fruits, but also hides the power to protect and revitalize your veins. The Hawthorn, or hawthorn, is that silent guardian, an unexpected ally in the fight against varicose veins. In this chapter, we will find out how this ancient plant can help you improve microcirculation and protect your veins.

Native to temperate regions of Europe, hawthorn has been revered for generations for its cardiotonic qualities. However, its benefits go beyond the heart, extending to the tiny veins that are part of our body's vast circulatory river.

It contains triterpene and phenolic acids, which reinforce its protective and repairing effects.

Benefits for Microcirculation

1. Relaxation glass:

What does this mean? Hawthorn promotes the secretion of nitric oxide, a crucial molecule that helps relax the smooth muscles in the veins. This facilitates freer blood flow and reduces pressure that can cause varicose veins.

2. Endothelial Protection:

How does it protect veins? The plant strengthens the internal barrier of the veins (the endothelium), inhibiting processes that can damage it and activating mechanisms that stabilize it. This is vital for preventing varicose veins, as a healthy endothelium prevents blood from pooling and forming varicose veins.

Clinical Use and Precautions

Therapeutic Applications: Hawthorn has shown promise in treating ischemia and preventing arrhythmias. Its ability to protect against reperfusion/ischemia injury makes it an ideal candidate for more in-depth studies in the context of venous diseases.

Adverse effects:

Although safe, some adverse effects such as dizziness and gastrointestinal discomfort have been reported. It is important to consult with a healthcare professional before starting any supplement, especially during pregnancy or breastfeeding.

Hawthorn, or hawthorn, has been researched for its ability to improve cardiovascular health and could benefit those with varicose veins for its effects on microcirculation. These compounds help dilate peripheral and coronary blood vessels, which improves blood flow to the heart and may be helpful in relieving associated conditions such as chest pain or angina.

In addition, Hawthorn promotes the secretion of nitric oxide, a natural vasodilator that relaxes blood vessels and improves overall circulation, which can be particularly beneficial for affected microcirculation in cases of varicose veins.

If you are considering including Hawthorn in your daily regimen, it is advisable to do so under medical supervision, especially if you are pregnant, breastfeeding, or taking heart disease medications, as it can interact with these treatments.

This natural approach, combined with an active lifestyle and healthy eating, can be a valuable part of your strategy to manage varicose veins and improve your cardiovascular well-being.

Practical Tips

Daily Addition: Consider including hawthorn in your daily regimen through capsules or teas. Make sure to use standardized extracts for the best results.

Combination of Treatments: Use hawthorn in combination with other varicose vein therapies, such as compression stockings and exercise, to maximize the beneficial effects.

How long does it take to see the effects of hawthorn?

The benefits of hawthorn can take several weeks to manifest. Persistence is key, and the effects can vary from person to person.

Are there any drug interactions with hawthorn?

Yes, hawthorn can interact with heart and blood pressure medications. Always consult with a healthcare professional before starting to take it, especially if you are already under medical treatment.

Tips for Medical Supervision

Regular Consultations: Before starting treatment with hawthorn, consult a healthcare professional. It is crucial to adjust the dose appropriately and monitor the response to treatment.

Monitoring Side Effects: Although hawthorn is safe, it is important to watch for side effects such as dizziness or gastrointestinal discomfort. Report any adverse symptoms to your doctor.

Conclusion: Beyond Beauty

Hawthorn is not only a beautiful plant; It is a testament to how nature provides us with powerful tools to take care of our health in a comprehensive way. By integrating Hawthorn into your life, you are not only choosing to treat your varicose veins, but you are also making a conscious decision to protect and improve your circulatory system.

Ginseng: An Ancient Ally for Modern Venous Health

Imagine for a moment a root that has not only been valued for millennia in traditional Asian medicine, but also possesses the power to revitalize your veins from within. We are talking about ginseng, a plant whose roots hide more than simple myths: they hide a natural pharmacy capable of significantly improving your venous circulation.

Discovering Ginseng

Revered in Eastern medicine for its ability to balance the body and mind, ginseng contains a number of bioactive compounds called ginsenosides. These compounds are responsible for many of ginseng's health benefits, and their study has fascinated doctors and scientists alike.

Bioactive Components and Their Effects

Ginsenosides (Rb1, Rg1, Rg3, Re, Rd): These saponins play a crucial role in promoting cardiovascular and venous health.

They act on the vascular system in ways that can transform the health of varicose vein sufferers.

Alkaloids and phenolic acids: They complement the action of ginsenosides, offering antioxidant and anti-inflammatory protection.

Benefits for Microcirculation

1. Vasodilation:

How does it work? Ginsenosides stimulate the production of nitric oxide in the endothelium, the inner layer of veins. This causes the vascular smooth muscles to relax, allowing the veins to dilate and facilitate better blood flow. Can you imagine facilitating the transit of blood through your veins like clearing a traffic jam on a busy road?

2. Endothelial Protection:

What does this imply? In addition to improving circulation, ginseng protects vein walls from reperfusion/ischemia (I/R) damage, which is when blood flow is restored to a previously oxygen-deprived area. This type of protection is crucial to preventing long-term venous damage.

Considerations and Adverse Effects

Although ginseng is a powerful ally for venous health, its use is not without precautions. Some adverse effects include nausea, diarrhea, and insomnia, and it is particularly important to avoid its consumption during pregnancy or breastfeeding due to its effects on myometrial tone and motility.

Have you ever considered how a plant like ginseng could alter the management of your varicose veins? What changes could you implement in your daily life to take advantage of its benefits?

Conclusion: Ginseng, more than a miraculous root

Ginseng offers more than anecdotes from traditional medicine; It offers solutions backed by modern science for contemporary circulatory problems. By integrating ginseng into your daily regimen, along with a balanced diet and exercise, you are not only taking care of your veins, but improving your overall vascular health.

In the following pages, we will continue to explore other natural remedies and nutritional strategies that complement the use of ginseng, ensuring that you have the necessary tools to live a life free from the limitations imposed by varicose veins.

Ginseng, prized in traditional Asian medicine for its many benefits, contains ginsenosides such as Rb1, Rg1, Rg3, Re, Rd, which are essential for improving cardiovascular and venous health. These compounds stimulate the production of nitric oxide, which facilitates vasodilation and improves microcirculation. In addition, ginseng offers antioxidant and anti-inflammatory protection, which is crucial for maintaining good vein health and preventing complications associated with varicose veins.

Benefits of Ginseng for Microcirculation and Venous Health

1. Vasodilation: Ginsenosides stimulate the relaxation of vascular smooth muscles, allowing for better blood flow and reducing pressure in the veins.

2. Endothelial Protection: Ginseng protects the endothelium, the inner layer of veins, from potential damage, which is vital for preventing long-term venous problems.

Adverse Effects and Precautions

Although ginseng is well-tolerated, it can cause nausea, diarrhea, and insomnia.

It is important to avoid consumption during pregnancy or breastfeeding due to its effects on myometrial tone and motility.

Practice

Integrating ginseng into your daily regimen could significantly improve your varicose vein management.

It is advisable to do so under medical supervision to adjust the dose appropriately and monitor possible adverse effects.

The use of ginseng, combined with a balanced diet and regular exercise, may offer a comprehensive strategy to improve vascular health and relieve varicose vein symptoms.

Practical Tips

Ginseng Incorporation: Integrate ginseng into your diet through ginseng capsules or tea. Be sure to start with low doses to assess tolerance.

Combination of Treatments: Combine the use of ginseng with other treatments recommended for varicose veins, such as leg elevations and the use of compression stockings, to optimize results.

How long should it take ginseng to see varicose veins improve?

Effects can vary, but it is recommended to evaluate the benefits after 8 to 12 weeks of consistent use.

Can ginseng interact with medications?

Yes, ginseng can interact with blood-thinning medications and those that affect the immune system. It is essential to consult with a doctor before starting ginseng, especially if you are already undergoing medical treatment.

Tips for Medical Supervision

Initial Consultation: Before starting ginseng supplementation, consult a healthcare professional to evaluate your specific situation and interactions with other treatments.

Response Monitoring: It is important to follow up regularly to adjust the dosage if necessary and monitor for any side effects or interactions with other medications you are taking.

Vitis vinifera L.: The Power of the Grapevine in the Fight Against Varicose Veins

In the heart of the vineyards, not only do the grapes that give rise to the world's most exquisite wines grow, but also a natural and powerful solution for those who suffer from varicose veins. Red Leaf Extract, derived from the Vitis vinifera L. plant, is an ally in vascular health thanks to its rich composition of bioactive compounds.

A Look at the Components of the Vine

The vine is not only the source of grapes, but also a reservoir of phenolic compounds such as resveratrol, gallic acid, catechin, and a variety of flavonoids and procyanidins. These components are known for their potent antioxidant and anti-inflammatory effects, which play a crucial role in protecting and improving microcirculation.

Key Benefits for Varicose Veins

1. Endothelial Protection and Vessel Relaxation:

How does it work? Resveratrol and procyanidins from grapevines can increase nitric oxide (NO) synthesis in the endothelium, which facilitates the relaxation of blood vessels and improves circulation. This effect is vital for preventing venous stasis, a predominant condition in varicose veins.

Visible Effects: Have you ever noticed a decrease in the heaviness and pain in your legs after a change in your diet or routine? These compounds help reduce those bothersome symptoms, significantly improving your quality of life.

2. Inflammation Reduction and Capillary Permeability:

Impact: Procyanidine B1 has anti-inflammatory effects that decrease capillary permeability. This process is critical for reducing edema and the feeling of heaviness in the legs, two common and debilitating symptoms of varicose veins.

Clinical Applications and Considerations

Clinical Use: Vitis vinifera L. has been effectively used in the treatment of peripheral venous disease and hemorrhoidal conditions. The reduction in vain diameter evidences its potential to improve venous condition.

Adverse Effects: Although well tolerated, it is important to be aware of possible gastrointestinal discomfort or allergic reactions. The inclusion of this extract should be carefully considered, especially if you are pregnant or breastfeeding.

Practical Implementation

Can you imagine integrating an element as natural as red leaf extract into your daily routine? Here are some suggestions:

Dietary Integration: Consider supplements containing Vitis vinifera L. extract, or incorporate natural products derived from the vine into your meals.

Medical Consultations: Do not forget to consult with your doctor before starting any supplementation, especially if you have pre-existing conditions.

As you walk through life, every step you take toward taking care of your veins is a step toward better health. Red Leaf Extract is not just a supplement; It is a testament to how nature can sustain and improve our vascular health.

Not only does this chapter give you an in-depth understanding of the benefits of Vitis vinifera L., but it also invites you to explore how you can make slight changes in your life for big improvements in your venous health. Are you ready to take that step?

It is important to note that although red leaf extract is well tolerated, it could cause gastrointestinal discomfort or allergic reactions in some cases. Therefore, it is recommended to discuss any supplementation with a healthcare professional, especially if you have pre-existing conditions or if you are pregnant or breastfeeding.

How long does it take for the effects of red vine extract on varicose veins to be seen?

The effects can vary, but it is recommended to evaluate the benefits after consistent use for at least 3 to 6 weeks.

Does red vine extract have side effects?

Although it is well tolerated, in some cases it can cause mild gastrointestinal discomfort. It is important to start with a low dose and gradually increase as tolerated.

Tips for Medical Supervision

Prior Evaluation: Before starting supplementation, a medical evaluation is crucial to ensure that there are no contraindications or risks of interactions with other medications.

Regular Follow-Up: Encourages regular follow-up with a healthcare professional to monitor response to treatment and adjust dosage if necessary.

Herbal Innovations in the Treatment of Venous Insufficiency

In this chapter we will explore how two powerful plants, Centella asiatica and Vitis vinifera, combined, are making their way into the treatment of chronic venous insufficiency, a condition that affects many people around the world and is related to the appearance of varicose veins.

Imagine for a moment two of the most powerful forces of nature in the field of phytotherapy joining their properties to offer an integrated and effective solution against varicose veins. Centella asiatica, known for its use in Ayurvedic and traditional Chinese medicine, and Vitis vinifera, better known as the grape plant, whose benefits transcend wine production, combine to form a formidable treatment.

1. Essential Recommendation:

The recommended ratio of Centella asiatica extract (EC) to Vitis vinifera extract (VVE) is 1:3. This combination has been shown, through rigorous studies, to be the most effective in reducing abnormal vascular permeability and inflammation, key aspects in the initial stages of venous insufficiency.

Inhibition of Inflammatory Meters:

The combined extracts have a significant effect on the reduction of inflammatory mediators such as nitric oxide and prostaglandin E2, key in the progression of pain and inflammation associated with varicose veins.

Modulation of the Nuclear Factor NF-κB:

By affecting the translocation of the transcription factor NF-κB, extracts modulate the expression of genes that promote inflammatory processes, thus providing significant relief from varicose vein symptoms.

Effective Reduction of Vascular Permeability:

Tests have shown that these combinations not only reduce inflammation, but also decrease vessel permeability, a crucial factor in reducing edema and improving patients' quality of life.

Practical Application and Recommendations

Incorporation into Treatment Plans:

Doctors can integrate these herbal combinations into a holistic treatment plan that includes both compression therapy and limb elevation measures, thereby optimizing therapeutic outcomes.

Dosage Monitoring and Adjustment:

It is vital that treatments are individually adjusted, and that continuous monitoring is conducted to ensure maximum efficacy and minimize potential side effects.

The combination of Centella asiatica and Vitis vinifera has been studied for its efficacy in reducing abnormal vascular permeability and inflammation, which are key aspects in the initial stages of chronic venous insufficiency. Studies suggest that the recommended ratio of Centella asiatica extract to Vitis vinifera extract is 1:3 to achieve effectiveness in the treatment of this condition.

The biological mechanisms involved include the inhibition of inflammatory mediators such as nitric oxide and prostaglandin E2, as well as the modulation of the nuclear factor NF-κB, which helps reduce inflammatory processes and vascular permeability. These combined effects can significantly decrease inflammation and edema in patients with varicose veins.

It is crucial that the implementation of this treatment is done under medical supervision to adjust the doses according to the patient's individual response and minimize side effects. In addition, it is recommended to integrate these herbal combinations into a larger treatment plan that may also include compression therapy and other measures to optimize therapeutic outcomes.

Since the combination of these plants presents itself as a promising and less invasive alternative for the treatment of chronic venous insufficiency, it is important for patients and healthcare providers to consider all available options, including natural treatments that may offer benefits without the risks associated with more invasive procedures.

Practical Tips

1. Start with Gradual Supplementation:

If you are considering starting with Centella Asiatica and Vitis vinifera supplements, start with a low dose and gradually increase based on tolerance and your healthcare professional's recommendations. This will help your body adjust to the treatment and allow you to detect side effects early.

2. Combine with Physical Therapies:

Integrate the use of these extracts with compression therapies and specific exercises for the legs. The combination of treatments can optimize outcomes and improve vein health holistically.

3. Keep a Symptom Diary:

Record your symptoms daily, any changes you notice and how you feel about taking the supplements. This will allow you to accurately track the effects of the treatment and discuss them with your doctor for necessary adjustments.

How long does it take for the combination of Centella asiatica and Vitis vinifera to work?

The effects may vary between individuals. Patients may notice improvements in symptoms of chronic venous insufficiency within the first 4 to 8 weeks of continuous use. It is important to be patient and consistent with supplementation.

Is it safe to take these supplements along with other medications?

While Centella asiatica and Vitis vinifera are safe, they can interact with other medications, especially blood thinners and anti-inflammatories. It is crucial to consult your doctor before starting supplementation to avoid adverse interactions.

Are there any side effects when using these supplements?

Side effects are rare, but may include mild gastrointestinal discomfort, dizziness, or allergic reactions. If you experience adverse effects, it is important to reduce the dose or discontinue use and consult a healthcare professional.

Tips for Medical Supervision

1. Initial Evaluation:

Perform a full medical evaluation before starting Centella Asiatica and Vitis vinifera supplements. This includes a physical exam and blood tests to establish a baseline of your venous and overall health.

This will help your doctor personalize your treatment and monitor the effects more accurately.

2. Regular Monitoring:

Schedule regular follow-up visits with your doctor to assess your progress and adjust doses if necessary. This will ensure that you get the maximum benefit from supplementation while minimizing any potential risks.

3. Symptom Report:

Tell your doctor about any changes in your symptoms, whether it is an improvement or a worsening. Details such as pain intensity, swelling, and any new discomfort should be reported. This will allow your doctor to adjust treatment effectively and in a timely manner.

Conclusion: A Promising Future

The combination of Centella asiatica and Vitis vinifera represents an exciting frontier in the treatment of varicose veins and venous insufficiency. Not only do these extracts offer a less invasive and more natural approach, but their potential to improve microcirculation and reduce inflammation opens new avenues to significantly improve the quality of life for those suffering from these conditions.

As we close this chapter, I invite you to reflect on how the integration of natural solutions can be a valuable complement or even an alternative to conventional methods, especially in the management of chronic conditions such as varicose veins. Are you ready to consider these natural options on your journey to better vascular health?

Witch Hazel Virginiana L. – A Natural Ally Against Varicose Veins

In our constant search for natural solutions to improve vascular health and combat varicose veins, we came across a valuable botanical resource: Hamamelis virginiana L., commonly known as witch hazel. This chapter delves into how witch hazel can be an effective adjunct in the management of varicose veins and other vascular conditions.

Have you ever wondered how a plant can significantly influence the health of your veins? Witch hazel is not only a popular ingredient in skincare products for its soothing effect, but it also possesses properties that can actively improve microcirculation and relieve the symptoms of varicose veins.

Composition and Action of Witch Hazel

Bioactive Constituents:

Witch hazel virginiana is composed of a rich amalgam of dyes, gallic acid, flavonoids such as catechins, saponins and essential oils that give it multiple therapeutic properties.

Benefits for Microcirculation:

Thanks to the tannins present, witch hazel offers astringent and hemostatic properties, essential for reducing superficial blood flow. This ability is particularly beneficial in the treatment of conditions such as dermatitis and peripheral venous disease (PVD), where skin integrity and underlying circulation are compromised.

Vasoconstriction and Inflammation Relief:

Acting as a natural vasoconstrictor, witch hazel improves venous tone by reducing vascular permeability and limiting inflammation, thanks to the inhibition of histamine release by its flavonoids.

Practice:

Although it is safe and well-tolerated, caution should be exercised when using it, especially in people with sensitive skin or those who are pregnant, due to the potential irritants and lack of extensive studies in these groups.

Practical Scenario and Usage Considerations

Imagine that you work from home, spending long hours in front of the computer. You notice heaviness and tiredness in your legs at the end of the day. Integrating witch hazel into your daily routine, through a gel or cream, could be a simple and effective method of relieving these symptoms. It would not only help improve circulation but also reduce any skin inflammation or irritation.

Witch hazel, scientifically known as Witch Hazel Virginiana, is a valuable resource for the management of varicose veins and other vascular conditions due to its bioactive components such as tannins, which give it astringent and hemostatic properties. These properties are especially useful for reducing surface blood flow and improving microcirculation, which is beneficial in the treatment of dermatitis and peripheral venous disease.

Although witch hazel is safe and well-tolerated when applied to the skin, there are potential side effects such as skin irritation, especially in people with sensitive skin. In addition, its use is not recommended during pregnancy or lactation due to the lack of data on its safety in these populations.

Clinical applications of witch hazel include its use in reducing inflammation and as a natural vasoconstrictor, which improves venous tone and limits inflammation by inhibiting the release of histamine by its flavonoids. This can be helpful in relieving symptoms related to varicose veins.

It is important that any integration of witch hazel into treatments for varicose veins or other medical conditions be discussed and supervised by a healthcare professional, to ensure proper and safe use.

Practical Tips

1. Regular Topical Application:

Apply witch hazel in the form of a gel or cream twice a day to the areas affected by varicose veins. This can help reduce inflammation, relieve itching, and improve microcirculation in the skin.

2. Use of Cold Compresses:

Use cold compresses soaked in witch hazel to reduce swelling and pain in your legs after extended periods of standing. Cold compresses can provide immediate relief and improve blood circulation.

3. Integration into the Skincare Routine:

Incorporate witch hazel into your daily skincare routine, especially if you experience skin irritation or inflammation related to varicose veins. Regular use can improve overall skin health and prevent varicose vein-related complications.

How does witch hazel work to improve vein health?

Witch hazel contains tannins, flavonoids, and essential oils that possess astringent and anti-inflammatory properties. These components help reduce blood vessel permeability and improve venous tone, which can relieve varicose vein symptoms such as swelling and pain.

Is it safe to use witch hazel during pregnancy?

Although witch hazel is safe for topical use, caution is advised during pregnancy due to the lack of extensive studies in this population. Always consult your doctor before starting any new treatment during pregnancy.

Can witch hazel cause side effects?

Topical use of witch hazel is well tolerated, but in some people, it may cause skin irritation or allergic reactions. If you experience redness, itching, or any other adverse reaction, discontinue use, and consult a healthcare professional.

Tips for Medical Supervision

1. Initial Evaluation:

Before you start using witch hazel, consult with a dermatologist to evaluate the severity of your varicose veins and determine the best way to incorporate witch hazel into your treatment. This ensures that you receive a personalized and safe treatment plan.

2. Regular Monitoring:

Schedule regular visits with your doctor to monitor the effectiveness of your witch hazel treatment and adjust as needed. Tracking allows you to quickly detect and manage any side effects or changes in the condition of your varicose veins.

3. Monitoring of Skin Reactions:

Tell your doctor about any adverse skin reactions when using witch hazel, such as irritation, redness, or itching. This allows you to adjust the treatment to minimize adverse effects and ensure the health of your skin.

Conclusion: A Remedy for All?

Throughout this chapter, we have explored how Witch Hazel can be an ally in the fight against varicose veins. Its ability to improve microcirculation and offer symptomatic relief makes it a valid option for those looking for natural alternatives. However, it is essential to consult a healthcare professional before starting any new treatment, especially if you are already under treatment for varicose veins or other medical conditions.

This chapter has not only brought you closer to the nature of this extraordinary plant but has also emphasized the importance of an individualized assessment and approach to the treatment of varicose veins. Are you ready to explore the benefits of witch hazel in your life?

Ginkgo Biloba L. – A Natural Reinforce-ment for the Venous System

At the heart of traditional and modern herbal medicine, we find the Ginkgo Biloba, an ancient tree that offers promising solutions for those facing varicose vein discomfort. This chapter explores how Ginkgo Biloba can be a valuable ally in venous health management, providing relief and improving the quality of life for those affected by this condition.

Did you know that Ginkgo Biloba is one of the living fossils of our flora? With a history dating back more than two hundred million years, this plant has not only survived climatic and geological changes but has also thrived. Its resistance makes it a symbol of longevity and, in medical terms, a source of bioactive components beneficial to our blood circulation.

Beneficial Mechanisms of Action:

Vasodilatory activity: Ginkgo promotes the expansion of blood vessels, thus facilitating better blood perfusion through the endothelium, the inner layer of blood vessels.

Endothelial Protection: Fights oxidative stress and decreases the adhesion of inflammatory molecules, helping to maintain the integrity of venous walls.

Specific Applications for People with Varicose Veins

Imagine feeling heaviness in your legs at the end of each day, a constant reminder of your varicose veins. Integrating Ginkgo Biloba into your regimen could significantly improve this symptom, thanks to its ability to improve microcirculation and facilitate more efficient venous return, thus relieving pressure in the veins.

Precautions and Practical Recommendations

Adverse effects to consider:

Although the benefits of Ginkgo are remarkable, it is wise to be on the lookout for potential side effects like bleeding complications, especially if you are taking blood-thinning medications.

Integration in Treatment:

Before starting any supplement, it is essential to consult with a medical professional. Ginkgo Biloba should be part of a comprehensive management plan that includes proper diet, exercise, and, if necessary, compression therapies.

Ginkgo Biloba, used for centuries in both traditional and modern medicine, offers beneficial properties for vascular health, particularly in the management of varicose veins.

Benefits and Mechanisms of Action

Vasodilation: Ginkgo Biloba promotes the expansion of blood vessels, thus improving blood perfusion through the endothelium. This action is beneficial in relieving symptoms such as heaviness in the legs caused by varicose veins.

Endothelial Protection: Fights oxidative stress and decreases the adhesion of inflammatory molecules, which is essential for maintaining the integrity of venous walls.

Precautions and Recommendations

Adverse Effects: Although Ginkgo Biloba is safe, it can cause bleeding complications, especially in combination with blood-thinning medications. Caution and medical consultation are recommended before starting any supplementation.

Integration into Treatment: Should be considered as part of a comprehensive management plan that includes diet, exercise, and compression therapies, if necessary. The commonly recommended dosage for circulatory benefits is 120 to 240 mg per day of standardized Ginkgo Biloba extract.

Conclusion

Ginkgo Biloba comes across as a valuable and potent resource for improving microcirculation and vascular health, which can be particularly helpful for people with varicose veins. Its use should be personalized and supervised by a health professional to ensure maximum efficacy and safety.

This chapter invites you to consider Ginkgo Biloba within a holistic approach to the treatment of varicose veins, highlighting the importance of careful evaluation and a personalized approach in the management of venous conditions.

Practical Tips

1. Dosage and Supplementation:

Start with a dose of 120 mg per day of standardized Ginkgo Biloba extract, divided into two daily doses. If necessary, you can increase the dose to 240 mg daily under medical supervision. Helps improve microcirculation and relieve symptoms of heaviness and pain in the legs.

2. Incorporation into the Daily Routine:

Integrate Ginkgo Biloba into your supplement regimen along with an antioxidant-rich diet and regular exercise to maximize its benefits. Enhances the effects of Ginkgo Biloba in improving vascular health and overall well-being.

3. Combine with Compression Therapies:

Wear compression stockings during the day to complement the use of Ginkgo Biloba and improve venous return. The combination of these therapies can offer more complete relief from varicose vein symptoms.

How does Ginkgo Biloba work to improve varicose veins?

Ginkgo Biloba improves microcirculation by promoting vasodilation and increasing blood flow through the endothelium. In addition, its antioxidant properties help protect the vein walls from oxidative damage.

Are there any side effects when using Ginkgo Biloba?

Although Ginkgo Biloba is safe, it can cause side effects such as headaches, dizziness, and gastrointestinal upset. It can also increase the risk of bleeding, especially in people who take blood thinners. It is essential to consult a doctor before starting supplementation.

Can I take Ginkgo Biloba if I am taking other medications?

Ginkgo Biloba can interact with several medications, including blood thinners, nonsteroidal anti-inflammatory drugs (NSAIDs), and certain antidepressants. Always consult your doctor before starting any new supplement to avoid adverse interactions.

Tips for Medical Supervision

1. Initial Evaluation:

Make an appointment with your doctor to assess the health of your veins and determine the proper dosage of Ginkgo Biloba. An accurate diagnosis and a personalized dose guarantee greater effectiveness and safety of the treatment.

2. Regular Monitoring:

Schedule regular appointments to monitor your response to treatment with Ginkgo Biloba and adjust the dosage if necessary. Regular monitoring allows any side effects or necessary adjustments to be detected and corrected in treatment.

3. Coagulation Tests:

If you are taking blood thinners, be sure to perform clotting tests regularly to monitor the risk of bleeding. This ensures that Ginkgo Biloba is safe to use and does not increase the risk of bleeding complications.

Conclusion: Ginkgo Biloba, A Natural Change for the Better?

Throughout this chapter, we have seen how Ginkgo Biloba not only symbolizes resilience and longevity, but also offers hope to those seeking natural relief from varicose veins. Its impact on microcirculation and vascular health makes it a valuable therapeutic option, which deserves consideration within a holistic treatment approach for venous insufficiency.

Do you feel ready to explore how this ancient, but always relevant, tree can help you manage your varicose vein symptoms? It is time to consider Ginkgo Biloba as part of your strategy for better vascular health.

Mangifera indica L. – A Tropical Ally in the Treatment of Varicose Veins

Have you ever wondered how something as delicious as mango can benefit your vascular health as well? In this chapter, we will explore how Mangifera indica L., better known as mango, becomes a crucial component for the management of varicose veins, thanks to its rich bioactive components and its beneficial effects on microcirculation.

Not only is mango tasty, but it is also loaded with a variety of health-promoting compounds:

Polyphenols: Mangiferin and procyanidins, known for their powerful antioxidant properties, stand out.

Hydroxybenzoic and Hydroxycinnamic Acids: Compounds such as gallic and ferulic acid, which offer anti-inflammatory and protective benefits for the endothelial cells in your veins.

Imagine that your veins are small rivers that need to flow freely to maintain the health of your circulatory system. The handle helps to:

Improve Reactive Hyperemia: Essential for an efficient vascular response to stress, which means your veins can better adapt to changes in blood flow, avoiding the stasis that leads to varicose veins.

Increase eNOS Expression: This is crucial for producing nitric oxide (NO), a vasodilator that relaxes veins, thereby improving circulation and reducing pressure that can cause varicose veins.

Mango not only improves blood flow; It acts at the cellular level to protect your veins:

Endothelial Enhancement: Increased production of NO by ginsenosides helps keep veins flexible and resilient.

Protection Against Postprandial Stress: Consuming mango can minimize vein damage after glucose-rich meals, a notable advantage for those looking to keep their veins healthy.

Dietary Mainstreaming: Add fresh mango to your salads, yogurts, or as a healthy snack between meals. Not only will you enjoy its taste, but also its circulatory benefits.

Medical Supervision: If you are considering mango supplements, especially if you have pre-existing medical conditions or are under pharmacological treatment, consult with your doctor first.

Mango offers more than an exotic flavor; It holds promise of improved vascular health and a more active, pain-free life for varicose vein sufferers. By integrating mango into your daily regimen, you are not only choosing to enjoy delicious fruit, but you are also taking an active step toward better vein health.

Would you dare to transform your diet and your health with the simple act of incorporating more mango into your meals? The time has come to see this tropical fruit in a whole new light, not just as a treat, but as part of your arsenal against varicose veins.

Practical Tips

1. Dietary Incorporation of Mango:

Add fresh mango to your daily meals. You can incorporate it into salads, smoothies, yogurts or simply as a healthy snack. Regular consumption of mango not only improves your vascular health thanks to its bioactive compounds, but also provides a healthy dose of essential vitamins and antioxidants.

2. Maintain a Balanced Diet:

Combine mango with other foods rich in antioxidants and anti-inflammatories such as red fruits, green leafy vegetables, and nuts. This combination enhances the beneficial effects of mango, improving the health of your veins and reducing the risk of inflammation and vascular damage.

3. Mango Supplements:

Consult your doctor about taking mango extract supplements, especially if you have pre-existing medical conditions. Supplements can be a concentrated and convenient way to get the benefits of mango, particularly if you cannot regularly consume it in your diet.

How can mango help in the prevention and management of varicose veins?

Mango contains polyphenols such as mangiferin and procyanidins, which have antioxidant and anti-inflammatory properties. These compounds help improve microcirculation and reduce inflammation, which can relieve varicose vein symptoms and prevent their progression.

Are there any side effects associated with excessive mango consumption?

Mango consumption is safe, but in excess it can cause diarrhea due to its high fiber content. In addition, people with latex allergy may experience allergic reactions due to the presence of similar substances in the handle.

Can I get the same benefits of mango through supplements?

Yes, mango extract supplements can provide a concentration of beneficial bioactive compounds. However, it is important to consult with a doctor before starting any supplement regimen to ensure its safety and effectiveness in your specific case.

Tips for Medical Supervision

1. Initial Consultation:

Before you start consuming mango regularly or taking mango supplements, talk to your doctor to assess your health status and receive personalized recommendations.

A doctor can help you determine the right amount and make sure there are no interactions with pre-existing medications or health conditions.

2. Continuous Monitoring:

If you decide to incorporate mango supplements, schedule regular appointments with your doctor to monitor your progress and adjust the dosage if necessary.

Continuous monitoring ensures that you are getting the desired benefits without adverse side effects.

3. Evaluation of Results:

Keep track of any changes in your varicose vein symptoms and share them with your doctor during appointments. This information will help your doctor evaluate the effectiveness of mango in your treatment and adjust optimize results.

Conclusion

Mango is not only a delicious fruit but also a powerful tool for improving vascular health and managing varicose veins. Its rich composition of polyphenols and other bioactive compounds makes it a valuable ally in the fight against varicose veins. By integrating mango into your diet and following your doctor's recommendations, you can take a significant step toward better vein health and a more active, pain-free lifestyle. Are you ready to make mango a regular part of your life and take advantage of all its benefits?

Vitamin B12 Essential for the Treatment of Varicose Veins

You may never have considered it, but what you eat can have a direct impact on the health of your veins. In this chapter, we will explore how proper nutrition, especially the balance of nutrients such as vitamin B12 and folic acid, can help manage and potentially improve conditions associated with varicose veins, including hyperhomocysteinemia (HHcy) which can complicate ulcer healing in people with varicose veins.

The Power of Nutrition in Vascular Health

Deficiency of key nutrients can not only affect your overall well-being, but it also plays a crucial role in vascular health. Let us see how:

1. Vitamin B12 in the Treatment of Ulcers and Varicose Veins:

Impact on Healing: Vitamin B12 is vital for cell regeneration and nerve function. Its deficiency has been significantly associated with the presence of diabetic foot ulcers (DFUs), a complication that can also affect those who suffer from varicose veins due to similar problems of poor circulation and neuropathy.

Specific Facts: Studies indicate that individuals with diabetes and low vitamin B12 have up to 3.1 times the risk of developing DFU. This data underscores the importance of monitoring and correcting this deficiency, especially in those who regularly consume metformin, a drug known to interfere with the absorption of vitamin B12.

Biological and Technical Mechanisms: How Vitamin B12 Works in Your Body

Nerve Function and Cell Regeneration: Vitamin B12 is essential for maintaining nerve cell integrity and blood cell formation. In the context of varicose veins, adequate availability of B12 helps prevent complications such as ulcers, which arise due to poor healing and peripheral neuropathy.

Important Interactions: It is crucial to be aware of the interactions between vitamin B12 and certain medications, such as metformin, commonly used in the treatment of diabetes. Medical supervision is essential to adjust supplementation appropriately and avoid deficiency.

Practical Recommendations to Incorporate into Your Life

Dietary Integration: Ensure adequate intake of vitamin B12 through foods rich in this nutrient, such as meats, eggs, and dairy products, or through supplements if a deficiency is detected.

Medical Monitoring and Supervision: Given the importance of vitamin B12 in vascular health and its interaction with medications, it is imperative to have regular medical follow-up to personalize supplementation and optimize nutrient levels in the body.

Conclusion: Nutrition as a Pillar of Vascular Health

To conclude this chapter is to recognize that the effective management of varicose veins goes beyond conventional treatment. Incorporating an informed nutritional approach, especially as it relates to vitamin B12 and other essential nutrients, can not only improve varicose vein-related symptoms, but also boost overall quality of life. Are you ready to make nutrition an integral part of your varicose vein management strategy?

Practical Tips

1. Natural Sources of Vitamin B12 and Folic Acid:

Incorporate foods rich in vitamin B12 such as red meat, fish, eggs, and dairy products. For folic acid, opt for leafy greens, legumes, and citrus fruits.

Not only do these foods improve your vascular health, but they also contribute to a balanced and nutritious diet.

2. Smart Supplementation:

If you are deficient in vitamin B12 or folic acid, consider supplementation under medical supervision. The recommended daily doses are 2.4 mcg of vitamin B12 and 400 mcg of folic acid for adults.

Proper supplementation can prevent and correct deficiencies, improving venous and overall health.

3. Regular Monitoring:

Perform regular blood tests to monitor vitamin B12 and folic acid levels, especially if you are being treated with medications such as metformin.

Maintaining optimal levels of these nutrients helps prevent vascular and neuropathic complications.

How does vitamin B12 affect the health of my veins?

Vitamin B12 is crucial for cell regeneration and nerve function. It helps maintain the integrity of endothelial cells in veins, which is essential for preventing complications such as venous ulcers.

What foods should I include in my diet to make sure I am getting enough vitamin B12 and folic acid?

Includes red meat, fish, eggs, and dairy products for vitamin B12. For folic acid, eat leafy greens, legumes, and citrus fruits.

Can I take vitamin B12 supplements if I am taking metformin?

Yes, but it is essential to do so under medical supervision. Metformin can interfere with the absorption of vitamin B12, so you may need to adjust the dose of the supplement.

Tips for Medical Supervision

1. Initial Consultation and Diagnosis:

Before starting any vitamin B12 or folic acid supplementation, make a medical consultation to evaluate your current levels through blood tests.

An accurate diagnosis allows you to customize supplementation to your specific needs, avoiding deficiencies and excesses.

2. Continuous Monitoring:

Schedule regular doctor visits to monitor your vitamin B12 and folic acid levels, especially if you are taking medications that interfere with their absorption, such as metformin.

Regular monitoring ensures that you maintain optimal nutrient levels, preventing complications and adjusting doses as needed.

3. Medication Adjustment:

If you are taking medications that affect the absorption of vitamin B12, such as metformin, discuss with your doctor whether to adjust your dose or change medications.

Tailoring your treatment to your nutritional needs helps improve your overall health and prevent problems related to vitamin deficiencies.

4. Risk Assessment:

If you have additional risk factors, such as diabetes or cardiovascular disease, make sure your doctor evaluates how these may influence your vitamin B12 and folic acid needs.

A complete risk assessment allows for a comprehensive approach to your treatment, addressing all complications and improving your quality of life.

5. Education and Ongoing Support:

Ask your doctor for educational information about the importance of vitamin B12 and folic acid in vascular health, as well as strategies for maintaining a balanced diet.

Being well-informed allows you to make better decisions about your health and maintain a lifestyle that supports the health of your veins.

How do I know if I am deficient in vitamin B12 or folic acid?

Common symptoms of vitamin B12 deficiency include fatigue, weakness, anemia, and neurological problems such as tingling in the extremities. Folic acid deficiency can cause anemia, irritability, and difficulty concentrating. A blood test is the best way to diagnose these deficiencies.

How quickly can I expect to see improvements in my varicose vein symptoms after I start taking vitamin B12 and folic acid?

Improvement times may vary depending on the level of deficiency and individual response to treatment. Some people may notice improvements in their energy levels and vein health within a few weeks, while for others it may take longer. It is important to follow your treatment plan and monitor your progress with your doctor.

Are there risks of taking too much vitamin B12 or folic acid?

Vitamin B12 is safe even in high doses, as the body eliminates excess through urine. However, too much folic acid can mask a vitamin B12 deficiency and lead to neurological problems. That is why it is crucial to follow your doctor's dosage recommendations and avoid unsupervised self-supplementation.

Incorporating vitamin B12 and folic acid into your diet and supplementation, under proper medical supervision, can significantly improve the health of your veins and the management of varicose veins. This nutritional approach not only addresses deficiencies that can complicate your condition, but also contributes to your overall well-being. Making informed decisions

and having the support of your doctor will allow you to optimize your treatment and enjoy a better quality of life.

The Power of Probiotics in Varicose Veins Management

Introduction: Is It Possible for Beneficial Microorganisms to Modify the Health of Your Veins?

You may have never thought about how the microorganisms that inhabit your gut can affect the health of your veins. In this chapter, we will explore an innovative approach to the management of varicose veins and their associated complications: probiotic supplementation. Join me on a journey through the science behind these little allies and how they could transform your fight against varicose veins.

Probiotics, those live microorganisms that when administered in adequate amounts confer benefits to the host's health, have shown promise not only in improving gut health but also in modulating inflammatory processes that affect other areas of the body, including the circulatory system.

1. Intervention and Clinical Outcomes:

Intervention Study: A group of participants received daily probiotics including Lactobacillus acidophilus, Lactobacillus casei, Lactobacillus fermentum, and Bifidobacterium bifidum for 12 weeks.

Observed Results: Significant reductions were recorded in venous ulcer dimensions—length, width, and depth—and improvements in general health indicators such as total cholesterol and levels of C-reactive protein (CRP), a marker of inflammation.

Underlying Biological Mechanisms

Probiotics work through several mechanisms that can be particularly beneficial for varicose vein sufferers:

Improved Gut Health and Reduced Systemic Inflammation: Probiotic supplementation strengthens the gut barrier, reduces the entry of toxins into the bloodstream, and modulates the immune system, decreasing systemic inflammation that can aggravate varicose veins.

Influence on Metabolism: By improving gut function, probiotics may also influence lipid and glucose metabolism, factors that affect vascular health.

Practical Applications: Integrating Probiotics into Your Daily Routine

Incorporation of Probiotics in the Diet: In addition to supplements, including foods rich in probiotics such as yogurts, kefir, sauerkraut, and other fermented foods can be an effective strategy to improve intestinal flora and, therefore, vascular health.

Medical Supervision: Before starting supplementation, especially if you are under medical treatment or have pre-existing conditions, it is crucial to consult with a healthcare professional. Monitoring ensures safe and effective integration of probiotics into your varicose vein treatment.

Adding probiotics to your health regimen can be a valuable approach not only to improve gut health but also to manage conditions such as varicose veins, offering an alternative or complement to conventional therapies. With their ability to reduce inflammation and improve circulation, probiotics are emerging as a fundamental component in the comprehensive management strategy of varicose veins.

In this chapter, we have explored how small, everyday choices in your diet and health management can have a profound impact on your vascular well-being. Are you ready to try probiotics and see how they can help you in your fight against varicose veins?

Available studies suggest that probiotics may improve gut health and reduce inflammation, which could indirectly benefit vascular health. In addition, it has been observed that they can influence lipid and glucose metabolism, which could also

126

positively impact varicose veins by improving circulation and reducing inflammation.

Despite the potential benefits, it is crucial to approach probiotic supplementation with caution, especially in people with pre-existing conditions or those who are under medical treatment, due to potential interactions and side effects. No specific interactions between probiotics and other medications have been documented in the context of varicose veins, but medical supervision is always recommended when introducing any new supplements, particularly in people taking blood-thinning medications or other complex treatments.

In summary, while the inclusion of probiotics in the treatment of varicose veins could offer some benefits due to their impact on inflammation and gut health, more clinical research is needed to establish firm and safe recommendations for their specific use in this condition.

Practical Tips

1. Incorporation of Foods Rich in Probiotics:

Add fermented foods such as yogurt, kefir, sauerkraut, and kimchi to your daily diet.

These foods are natural sources of probiotics that can help balance your gut flora and improve your vascular health by reducing inflammation.

2. Probiotic supplementation:

If you decide to take probiotic supplements, look for those that contain strains such as Lactobacillus acidophilus, Lactobacillus casei, Lactobacillus fermentum, and Bifidobacterium bifidum.

These strains have been shown to have beneficial effects in reducing inflammatory markers and improving overall health.

3. Consistency in Consumption:

For maximum benefits, consume probiotic-rich foods or supplements regularly and consistently.

Regular consumption helps maintain a balanced gut flora and reduced inflammation, which is crucial for vascular health.

How do I know if I need probiotics?

If you experience frequent digestive problems, inflammation, or have a history of long-term antibiotic use, you may benefit from probiotics. However, it is important to talk to your doctor to assess your specific situation.

Can probiotics really improve my varicose veins?

Although specific studies on probiotics and varicose veins are limited, evidence suggests that probiotics may reduce systemic inflammation and improve gut health, which may indirectly benefit vascular health and aid in the management of varicose veins.

Are there any side effects when taking probiotics?

In general, probiotics are safe for most people. Some may experience mild digestive symptoms such as bloating or gas at the onset of consumption, which usually disappear after a few days. It is crucial to start with low doses and gradually increase them.

Tips for Medical Supervision

1. Initial Consultation and Diagnosis:

Before starting probiotic supplementation, make a medical consultation to assess your specific needs.

An accurate diagnosis ensures that you receive the right type and number of probiotics for your specific situation.

2. Continuous Monitoring:

Schedule regular doctor visits to monitor the effects of probiotics on your vascular health.

Regular follow-up allows supplementation to be adjusted as needed to maximize benefits and minimize any adverse effects.

3. Drug Interactions:

Tell your doctor about any medications you are taking to evaluate potential interactions with probiotics.

This is especially important if you are taking antibiotics or immunosuppressive medications, as these can interact with probiotics.

Adding probiotics to your health regimen can be a valuable approach not only to improve gut health but also to manage conditions such as varicose veins, offering an alternative or complement to conventional therapies. With their ability to reduce inflammation and improve circulation, probiotics are emerging as a fundamental component in the comprehensive management strategy of varicose veins.

Gratitude

I want to express my sincere thanks to all the people who have purchased this book with the purpose of learning more about the management of varicose veins through nutrition and natural therapies. Your trust in this project means a lot to me and I hope that the information presented here will be of immense help to you on your path to better health.

To those who face the challenges of varicose veins daily, I want to say that I admire your determination and effort to improve your quality of life. This book is written for you, in hopes of offering you relief and effective solutions.

If you have found the content of this publication valuable, I invite you to leave your comments and suggestions on topics that you would like to see in future books. Also, if you have a moment, it would be an immense help to me if you shared your opinion and rated this book in the store where you purchased it. Your support will help more people discover my work and motivate me to continue producing books on relevant and useful topics in the field of health and nutrition.

Always remember that a proper diet and a comprehensive approach can prevent and treat many health problems, including varicose veins. Thank you again for your support and for being part of this community dedicated to wellness and health. Together we can achieve a healthier, hassle-free life!

Thank you!

Bibliography:

1.   Melo PG, Mota JF, Nunes CAB, et al. Effects of Oral Nutritional Supplementation on Patients with Venous Ulcers: A Clinical Trial. J Clin Med. 2022;11(19):5683. Published 2022 Sep 26. doi:10.3390/jcm11195683

2.   Takai Y, Hiramoto K, Nishimura Y, Uchida R, Nishida K, Ooi K. Association between itching and the serum zinc levels in patients with varicose veins. J Pharm Health Care Sci. 2017;3:24. Published 2017 Sep 21. doi:10.1186/s40780-017-0092-9

3.   Nocera R, Eletto D, Santoro V, et al. Design of an Herbal Preparation Composed by a Combination of Ruscus aculeatus L. and Vitis vinifera L. Extracts, Magnolol and Diosmetin to Address Chronic Venous Diseases through an Anti-Inflammatory Effect and AP-1 Modulation. Plants (Basel). 2023;12(5):1051. Published 2023 Feb 26. doi:10.3390/plants12051051

4.   Raposo A, Saraiva A, Ramos F, et al. The Role of Food Supplementation in Microcirculation-A Comprehensive Review [published correction appears in Biology (Basel). 2023 Sep 01;12(9):1198. doi: 10.3390/biology12091198]. Biology (Basel). 2021;10(7):616. Published 2021 Jul 2. doi:10.3390/biology10070616

5.   Qiu Y, Osadnik CR, Team V, Weller CD. Effects of physical activity as an adjunct treatment on healing outcomes and recurrence of venous leg ulcers: A scoping review. Wound Repair Regen. 2022;30(2):172-185. doi:10.1111/wrr.12995

6.   Bossart S, Boesch PF, Keo HH, Staub D, Uthoff H. Endovenous Thermal Ablation for Treatment of Symptomatic Saphenous Veins-Does the Body Weight Matter?. J Clin Med.

2023;12(17):5438. Published 2023 Aug 22. doi:10.3390/jcm12175438

7. Bechara N, Gunton JE, Flood V, Hng TM, McGloin C. Associations between Nutrients and Foot Ulceration in Diabetes: A Systematic Review. Nutrients. 2021;13(8):2576. Published 2021 Jul 27. doi:10.3390/nu13082576

www.ingramcontent.com/pod-product-compliance
Lightning Source LLC
Chambersburg PA
CBHW071027250726
48653CB00005B/1743